Ehlers-Danlos S

A Beginner's 3-Step Plan to Managing EDS Through Diet and Other Natural Methods, With Sample Recipes

Disclaimer

By reading this disclaimer, you are accepting the terms of the disclaimer in full. If you disagree with this disclaimer, please do not read the guide.

All of the content within this guide is provided for informational and educational purposes only, and should not be accepted as independent medical or other professional advice. The author is not a doctor, physician, nurse, mental health provider, or registered nutritionist/dietician. Therefore, using and reading this guide does not establish any form of a physician-patient relationship.

Always consult with a physician or another qualified health provider with any issues or questions you might have regarding any sort of medical condition. Do not ever disregard any qualified professional medical advice or delay seeking that advice because of anything you have read in this guide. The information in this guide is not intended to be any sort of medical advice and should not be used in lieu of any medical advice by a licensed and qualified medical professional.

The information in this guide has been compiled from a variety of known sources. However, the author cannot attest to or guarantee the accuracy of each source and thus should not be held liable for any errors or omissions.

You acknowledge that the publisher of this guide will not be held liable for any loss or damage of any kind incurred as a result of this guide or the reliance on any information provided within this guide. You acknowledge and agree that you assume all risk and responsibility for any action you undertake in response to the information in this guide.

Using this guide does not guarantee any particular result (e.g., weight loss or a cure). By reading this guide, you acknowledge that there are no guarantees to any specific outcome or results you can expect.

All product names, diet plans, or names used in this guide are for identification purposes only and are the property of their respective owners. The use of these names does not imply endorsement. All other trademarks cited herein are the property of their respective owners.

Where applicable, this guide is not intended to be a substitute for the original work of this diet plan and is, at most, a supplement to the original work for this diet plan and never a direct substitute. This guide is a personal expression of the facts of that diet plan.

Where applicable, persons shown in the cover images are stock photography models and the publisher has obtained the rights to use the images through license agreements with third-party stock image companies.

Introduction

Ehlers-Danlos Syndrome (EDS) is a group of disorders that affect connective tissues. Connective tissues are proteins that support the skin, bones, and joints. EDS can cause joint dislocations and fragile skin and tissue.

There are different types of EDS, each with its own set of symptoms. The most common type is hypermobile EDS (hEDS), which is marked by increased joint flexibility and fragile skin. Symptoms usually affect each person differently, so there isn't a template solution or treatment for everyone.

There is no cure for EDS, but treatments can help manage symptoms. In severe cases, joint dislocations may require surgery to prevent further damage. However, this doesn't mean you can't enjoy life to the fullest. There are different ways you can manage EDS at home, with the guidance of your doctor and your family. You can still enjoy life to the fullest by choosing what's best for you.

In this beginner's quick start guide, you will discover:
• All about Ehler-Danlos Syndrome
• EDS symptoms and causes
• How EDS is diagnosed and treated
• Different ways to manage EDS
• Following an EDS-friendly diet

What Is Ehlers-Danlos Syndrome?

Ehlers-Danlos Syndrome (EDS) is a group of disorders that affect connective tissues. Connective tissues are proteins that support the skin, bones, and joints. For example, collagen is a type of connective tissue that gives skin elasticity. Collagen is also found in tendons, which connect muscles to bones, and in ligaments, which connect bones to other bones. Because EDS can cause problems with these tissues, it can result in joint dislocations and fragile skin and tissue.

EDS can cause joint dislocations and fragile skin and tissue. There are different types of EDS, each with its own set of symptoms. The most common type is hypermobile EDS (hEDS), which is marked by increased joint flexibility and fragile skin. For example, people with hEDS may be able to extend their joints further than people without the condition. This increased flexibility can lead to joint pain and dislocations. Joints may pop out of place (dislocate) easily or with little force.

Skin in people with hEDS is often thin and elastic. This can cause it to tear or bruise easily. The skin may also feel stretched or "paper-like." It's not unusual for people with hEDS to develop stretch marks in areas where the skin has been stretched, such as during pregnancy.

Another type of EDS, called vascular EDS (vEDS), is the most severe form of the condition. It is marked by thin, fragile skin that tears or bruises easily. People with vEDS are also at risk for rupturing (tearing) arteries, veins, or organs. This can lead to life-threatening internal bleeding.

Some other types of EDS include:
• kyphoscoliotic EDS (kEDS): This form of EDS is marked by severe curvature of the spine and fragile skin.
• arthrochalasia dysplasia (aEDS): This form is characterized by loose joints and thin, fragile skin.
• dermatosparaxis EDS (dEDS): This form is characterized by very fragile skin that sags and forms wrinkles easily.
• Brittle cornea syndrome (BCS): This form of EDS is marked by thin, fragile corneas (the clear outer layer of the eye) that are at risk for rupturing.

Symptoms of EDS
The symptoms of EDS vary depending on the type of disorder. They can range from mild to severe. Some people with EDS have only a few symptoms, while others are more severely affected.

Common symptoms of EDS include:
• Joint pain. These can be caused by joint dislocations or by stretched or torn ligaments and tendons.
• Joint dislocation. This can occur with little or no trauma. The joints may pop out of place (dislocate) easily or with little force.

- Skin problems. These can include thin, elastic skin that bruises easily, stretch marks, and slow healing wounds.
- Digestive problems. These can include gastroesophageal reflux disease (GERD), abdominal pain, and bloating.
- Fatigue. This can be caused by poor sleep or by chronic pain.

Causes

The cause of most types of EDS is unknown. However, it is thought to be caused by a mutation in a gene that helps produce collagen or other connective tissues. These genes are passed down from parents to children. In some cases, the gene mutation occurs spontaneously (without being passed down from a parent). The mutation causes the body to produce defective collagen or other connective tissues. This can result in joint instability, fragile skin, and other symptoms of EDS.

Most types of EDS are hereditary, meaning they are passed down from parents to children. In some cases, the gene mutation that causes EDS occurs spontaneously (without being passed down from a parent). This is called a de novo mutation.

There are several different genes that have been linked to EDS. Mutations in any of these genes can cause the condition. The most common gene linked to EDS is COL5A1. This gene provides instructions for making type V collagen, which is found in tendons and ligaments. Mutations in COL5A1 can cause different types of EDS, including classical EDS, hypermobile EDS, and vascular EDS.

Other genes that have been linked to EDS include:
- COL3A1
- TNXB
- PLOD1
- CHST14

Mutations in these genes can cause different types of EDS, including classical EDS, kyphoscoliotic EDS, brachydactyly type EDS, and spondylodysplasia EDS.

Ehlers-Danlos syndrome occurs in both males and females. The condition is estimated to affect 1 in every 5,000 people worldwide.

Diagnosing and Treating EDS

In diagnosing and treating EDS, the medical history of your family will be reviewed by your doctor

Diagnosis
Ehlers-Danlos syndrome can be difficult to diagnose because the symptoms vary widely from person to person. There is no single test that can diagnose the condition.

Instead, your doctor will use a combination of tests and procedures to make the diagnosis. These may include blood tests to check for genes linked to EDS; imaging tests such as X-rays, CT scans, or MRIs to look for joint damage; and skin biopsies to examine collagen fibers in the skin.

X-rays are simply pictures of bones. A CT scan uses a series of X-rays and computer technology to show detailed pictures of tissues inside the body. An MRI also uses magnetic fields and radio waves, as well as computer image processing, to create a detailed view of soft tissues such as ligaments, tendons, and blood vessels.

One example of a skin biopsy that can be used to diagnose EDS is the Ghent nosology. This involves taking a small sample of skin and examining it under a microscope. The sample is then graded on a scale from I to VI, with I being the mildest form and VI being the most severe. Typically, someone with EDS will have a skin biopsy that falls somewhere in the middle of this scale.

Another test that can be used to diagnose EDS is a skin punch biopsy. In this procedure, a small sample of skin is removed using a special needle with a circular tip. The skin sample is then sent to a laboratory to be examined under a microscope.

The difference between the two biopsies is that with a skin punch biopsy, the entire sample is sent to a laboratory for examination. With the Ghent nosology, only part of the sample is examined under a microscope by a medical professional in a clinic or hospital setting.

Either test can be used to diagnose EDS and help determine which type of disorder a person has.

Treatment
There is no cure for Ehlers-Danlos syndrome. However, treatment can help relieve some of the symptoms and prevent complications from developing, such as joint dislocations and early onset arthritis.

Treatments may include:
● Physical therapy to improve joint function and flexibility
● Orthopedic bracing or splinting to help stabilize the joints

• Occupational therapy to teach you exercises and techniques to use in daily activities, such as dressing and bathing
• Medications to manage chronic pain or other symptoms of EDS, such as osteoarthritis.

Typically, treatment for EDS focuses on managing the symptoms and preventing complications from developing. This may involve physical therapy to improve joint function, occupational therapy to learn exercises and techniques for daily activities, and medications to manage pain or other symptoms of the condition.

Natural Ways to Manage Ehlers-Danlos Syndrome

In addition to conventional treatments for Ehlers-Danlos syndrome, there are several natural methods that may help manage the condition.

There are a variety of different treatments that can be used to manage the symptoms of Ehlers Danlos Syndrome

● Regular exercise, including stretching and low-impact activities like walking or swimming

The reason why exercise is so beneficial for managing the symptoms of EDS is that it can help improve flexibility and joint function, reduce pain, and prevent complications from developing.

To get started, it's important to consult with a physical therapist or other healthcare professional to create an exercise plan that's tailored to your needs.

● Massage therapy to help relieve pain and improve circulation

Massage therapy is a popular natural treatment for pain relief. It can also help improve circulation, which is essential for healing.

There are a number of reasons why massage therapy can be an effective treatment for various conditions. For one, massage can help to relax the muscles and reduce tension in the body. This can help to relieve pain and improve the range of motion. Additionally, massage can increase circulation and promote healing by increasing blood flow to the affected area. Finally, massage can also help to reduce stress and promote relaxation. These factors all combine to make massage therapy a valuable treatment for certain conditions.

One of the main reasons why massage therapy is effective for treating many conditions is because it can help to reduce tension and relieve pain in the muscles. This can be especially beneficial for those suffering from chronic muscle pain, as it can help to decrease inflammation and relax the affected area. In addition, massage has also been shown to improve range of motion by relaxing tight muscles and releasing any tension that may be restricting movement.

Another reason why massage therapy works so well is that it helps to increase circulation throughout the body, which promotes healing and can reduce pain. When the muscles are relaxed and the circulation is increased, more oxygen and nutrients can be delivered to the affected area, which can speed up the healing process. Additionally, massage therapy can also help to reduce stress, which can often contribute to pain and discomfort. By promoting relaxation, massage therapy can help to ease both physical and emotional symptoms.

Massage therapy is a safe and effective treatment for many conditions, and it can offer a number of benefits for those suffering from pain or stress. If you are considering massage therapy as a treatment option, be sure to discuss it with your doctor first to ensure that it is appropriate for your individual needs.

● Stress management techniques, such as yoga, deep breathing exercises, or meditation

Studies have shown that there is a link between stress and chronic pain. Therefore, managing stress can help reduce pain levels. According to the British Journal of Psychiatry, individuals with hypermobility issues are up to 16 times more represented than those with anxiety disorders.

There are a number of ways that you can manage stress in your life. Here are some tips to help you get started:

1. Identify the sources of your stress.
What are the things in your life that tend to cause you to stress? Once you know what these things are, you can start to take steps to avoid them or deal with them in a better way.

2. Make time for relaxation and fun.
It's important to have some time each day where you can relax and enjoy yourself. This can help reduce the overall amount of stress in your life.

3. Seek professional support if necessary.
If your stress is getting out of control, it may be helpful to talk to a mental health professional or other trusted professional for guidance on how to better manage it. With the right tools and strategies, you can learn how to effectively manage stress in your life no matter what challenges come your way.

4. Get enough sleep.
Sleep is crucial for overall well-being and can help you manage stress levels. Make sure to get an adequate amount of sleep each night so you can feel rested

The Ehlers-Danlos Syndrome diet

Another helpful way to manage Ehlers-Danlos syndrome is through diet. While there's no specific "Ehlers-Danlos Syndrome Diet," eating a healthy, well-balanced diet that includes plenty of fruits, vegetables, and whole grains is essential. It's also important to get adequate sleep and rest, as well as to reduce stress as much as possible.

Foods to Eat Less Of

There are a few foods that should be avoided or eaten in moderation if you have Ehlers-Danlos syndrome. These include:

• Processed foods, especially those that contain high levels of salt, sugar, and unhealthy fats

Processed foods are defined as "foods that have been changed from their natural state, either by canning, preserving, freezing, or dehydration." In other words, foods that have been altered in some way before being sold to consumers. This can include adding or removing certain ingredients, or changing the physical form of the food.

Processed foods are often criticized for being unhealthy, as they may contain high levels of sugar, fat, and salt. They may also be lacking in important nutrients like fiber and vitamins. However, not all processed foods are bad for you. Some processing methods can actually improve the nutritional value of foods, and make them easier to store and transport.

• Dairy products, particularly those that contain casein or gluten, which may cause inflammation or trigger allergic reactions

Gluten is a type of protein found in wheat, barley, and rye. For some people, gluten can cause inflammation or trigger an immune reaction. This can lead to symptoms such as bloating, diarrhea, fatigue, and headaches.

Casein is a type of protein found in milk and other dairy products. Like gluten, casein can cause inflammation or trigger an immune reaction in some people. This can lead to symptoms such as bloating, diarrhea, fatigue, and headaches.

• Saturated fat, which is usually found in red meat, full-fat dairy, and other high-fat foods

Saturated fats are a type of fat found in some animal products and tropical oils. The structure of saturated fats allows them to be solid at room temperature. Saturated fats are found in larger quantities in foods such as butter, cheese, and red meat.

While saturated fats are not necessary for good health, they can have negative effects on cholesterol levels and heart health if consumed in excess. Too much saturated fat can raise LDL (bad) cholesterol levels, which can lead to heart disease. Therefore, it is important to limit the amount of saturated fat you consume.

These fats are not good for people with EDS because they may increase inflammation and lead to other health problems. Therefore, it is important to limit or avoid foods that contain saturated fats if you have Ehlers-Danlos syndrome.

Healthy alternatives to foods high in saturated fat include leaner meats, low-fat dairy products, and vegetable oils. When cooking with saturated fats, it is also important to use moderate heat to avoid damaging the fat molecules.

Foods to Eat More Of
Typical to most diet plans, eating healthy foods is always the best advice. However, as there may be restrictions with regard to specific conditions connected to EDS, or at least with the various symptoms that affect the person with EDS, checking the food you need to consume is just as important as refraining from the food you need to eat less.

● Fruits and vegetables that are high in fiber to help with digestion.

These fruits and vegetables are also rich in many other nutrients that have great health benefits. For example, apples contain a compound called quercetin which is thought to have anti-inflammatory effects. Additionally, the fiber found in these foods can lower cholesterol levels and help reduce the risk of heart disease. Overall, incorporating more fruits and vegetables into your diet is an excellent way to improve overall health and maintain a healthy weight.

Some other fruits you can include are the following:
- apples
- pears
- prunes
- berries
- peas
- lentils
- beans

- Omega-3 fats are essential fat that people need for normal physiological function. Human beings cannot live without them. In fact, every single cell in our bodies needs omega-3 fats for proper functioning.

Some examples of omega-3 fats include eicosapentaenoic acid (EPA) and docosahexaenoic acid (DHA). These are found naturally in foods like fatty fish, nuts, and seeds. In addition to supporting normal bodily function, omega-3 fats also play an important role in brain health.

Here are some foods that contain omega-3 fats:
- salmon
- tuna
- mackerel
- herring
- anchovies

- sardines
- flaxseeds
- chia seeds
- walnuts

You can also get omega-3 fats from supplements. Fish oil supplements are a good source of EPA and DHA. These supplements can be especially beneficial for people who do not eat fish or other seafood regularly.

- Legumes are a type of plant that includes beans, lentils, and peas. Legumes are an excellent source of protein, fiber, and many other nutrients. They are also low in fat and calories.

Some examples of legumes include black beans, kidney beans, lentils, chickpeas, and soybeans. These foods can be eaten cooked or raw. Legumes can also be made into flour or used as a vegan meat replacement.

All About Responsible Eating
As mentioned above, there isn't exactly a diet that's specifically designed for this condition. What you'll most likely end up doing is curating your own meal plans that will only use ingredients that are highly recommended for your consumption.

Make sure that before anything else, you consult first with your doctor so they can be made aware of your desire and intention to manage your condition by your own means and in the comforts of your own home. This is actually important because it's best to start a diet program where you understand the importance of each food item in your diet, and how each can help you and affect your health. This way your doctor can also help you curate your own food lists dos and don'ts.

Another thing to remember is that EDS symptoms for each patient are different, so what applies to you may not be wholly applicable to another. The possibility of complications and other conditions, linked or not to EDS, can also be taken into consideration when talking to a professional health provider. This is why it's good to always inform your doctor first before doing anything.

Don't forget your goal for doing this diet—it's to help manage your condition. It's expected that if the diet works out well for you, you will start to see an improvement in your overall well-being. You may also start to lose weight or feel lighter. You may also start to feel more energetic and positive. These are just some of the other things that may improve when you become more responsible for what you consume.

7-Day Meal Plan

Here is a sample meal plan you can follow or modify to use either weekly or monthly. It's best to make a meal plan earlier so that you can purchase ingredients beforehand.

	Breakfast	Lunch	Dinner
Day 1	Spinach Omelet	Greek Salad with Arugula	Seared Salmon
Day 2	Cherry-Coconut Porridge	Mediterranean Tuna Salad	Squash and Spinach Medley
Day 3	Bean Soup and Greens	Barley and Chicken Soup	Salmon Salad
Day 4	Cherry-Coconut Porridge	Grilled Eggplant Salad	Chicken Seafood Paella
Day 5	Spinach Omelet	Black Beans and Rice	Cod Burger
Day 6	Chia Seed and Strawberry Pudding	Salmon Salad	Barley and Chicken Soup
Day 7	Squash and Spinach Medley	Avocado and Tuna Salad	Chicken Seafood Paella

3-Step Plan diet to Manage Ehlers-Danlos Syndrome

Now that you know more about Ehlers-Danlos syndrome and what foods to eat or avoid, you may be wondering how to put this information into action. Here is a 3-step plan to help you make dietary changes that will improve your symptoms:

Step 1 – Keep a food diary
Keeping a food diary is just as simple as it sounds. It's where you watch out for your meal plans for, say, a week or a month. You may also include here your food lists of dos and don'ts.

Generally, a food diary is where you document all the food you eat during your diet program. You write them down in columns including one where you'll take note of what you feel or experience after the meal. While it may either seem tedious or pointless at first, don't skip your food diary. Documenting what you eat and how you feel about them will help you understand better just how the food you eat generally affects you.

At the same time, keeping a diary can also help you curate your meal plans better in the future. During your next doctor's appointment after your, say one-week diet, present the result of your food diary to your doctor so you both can discuss why and how those food items made you feel or experience that way and perhaps even tweak your food list and your future meal plans.

Here's a sample food diary template you can copy or modify:

Day - Time of meal	Food (Ingredients)	Serving	Notes/Remarks
Wednesday Lunch	Meal name	1	I feel full after only one serving.
Wednesday Dinner	Meal name	1	I think it's best to replace one ingredient with the other.
Thursday Breakfast	Meal name	1	My stomach ached after eating

Step 2 – Stay active and do therapy

Exercising and staying active are activities that greatly benefit almost everyone. Different brain chemicals that benefit the body and mind are released when you exercise and do recreational activities that invigorate the body. Exercising also helps the mind relax and uplifts the mood.

There are these exercises that help the muscle and bones to stretch and strengthen, which releases tension and eventually help the body to relax. Doing light exercises such as walking, swimming, or just consistently staying active will definitely help in improving your body. If you are able to move around more comfortably, it'll of course be beneficial to you.

If you plan to do simple walking exercises or try other kinds of light exercises, make sure you inform your doctor about it. If you were recommended to follow a specific exercise and fitness plan, make sure that you follow that plan your therapist made for you. But even at home, doing menial and light chores is also a form of staying active. Just try to avoid always sitting or lying down if possible.

Usually, staying active becomes a much easier task when you have someone doing it with you. It's best if your family and friends can join you in doing these activities. Even brisk walking with a companion from time to time is much more motivating than doing it alone all the time.

Step 3 – Learn to manage stress
Stress is inevitable in everyone's life. However, that doesn't mean it cannot be managed. There are different ways to manage and cope with stress, and understanding what works for you will surely be helpful.

When you are in a stressful situation, make sure that you're able to stay calm and keep a clear mind. Take deep breaths and try not to panic or overthink. If you need the feel to vent out or talk to someone about your stress, don't hesitate to reach out to your support group. The goal isn't always to find a solution to the problem, sometimes just talking about it helps relieve stress.

See also if there are other recreational activities that can help you blow off your steam. For some, coloring or painting helps them relax and clear their mind. Others find that nature walks calm them down. Others find that crocheting, writing, or even listening to music relieves their stress. If you have these types of hobbies that help you put your mind off of things, go ahead and do them.

Exercising is also a great way to release stress. That's why it's highly encouraged for you to stay active even if it means only doing light exercises or doing light tasks around the house. According to studies, exercising truly does help relieve stress that lasts for a long time. You also end up having a clearer and better mindset, which will greatly affect your mood, judgment, and decision-making.

Sample Recipes

Greek Salad with Arugula

Ingredients:
- 1-1/2 lbs. or 750 g sweet potatoes, washed well
- salt, preferably Greek sea salt
- 1 large red onion or a bunch of scallions, sliced thinly
- 2 bunches of fresh arugula, coarsely chopped
- 1/2 virgin Greek olive oil
- 3-4 tbsp. red wine vinegar

Instructions:
1. Place sweet potatoes in a large pot with cold salted water. Bring to a boil over medium heat.
2. Reduce heat to low and simmer for about 15 minutes.
3. Remove, cool slightly, peel, and cut into bite-sized chunks.
4. Transfer to a serving bowl.
5. Place the arugula and onions or scallions in the bowl with the sweet potatoes.
6. Season with salt. Toss with olive oil and vinegar.
7. If desired, add crumbled feta or goat's milk cheese.
8. Serve immediately.

Salmon Salad

Ingredients:
- 2 large filets of wild salmon, either poached or grilled and then chilled
- 1 cup cherry tomatoes, halved
- 2 red onions, sliced
- 1 tbsp. balsamic vinegar
- 1 tbsp. capers
- 1 tbsp. fresh dill, finely chopped
- 1 tbsp. extra-virgin olive oil
- 1/4 tsp. pepper, freshly ground
- salt

Instructions:
1. Remove skin and bones from the cooled salmon.
2. Break salmon into chunks, and place them into a bowl.
3. Add tomatoes, red onion, and capers. Toss ingredients.
4. Combine balsamic vinegar, olive oil, and dill in a separate bowl.
5. Pour the mixture over salmon chunks. Toss again.
6. Sprinkle it with salt and pepper to taste.
7. Chill salad for at least half an hour before serving.

Avocado and Tuna Salad

Ingredients:
- 2 whole avocado fruits, slightly crushed
- 1/2 cup of pecans
- 1 cup of steamed and cubed chicken breast
- 1 cup of tuna in oil
- salt, to taste
- pepper, to taste

Instructions:
1. Mix all ingredients in a large bowl.
2. Add a dash of salt and pepper to taste.
3. Chill for at least an hour before serving.

Seared Salmon

Ingredients:
- 1-1/2 tbsp. canola oil
- 4 pcs. salmon filets, each filet about 1-inch thick
- 1 tsp. kosher salt
- 1 tsp. ground black pepper, 1 teaspoon
- 2/3 cups shallots, thinly sliced, 2/3 cup
- 3 cups cherry tomatoes, 3 cups
- 2 tbsp. balsamic vinegar
- 1/2 cup basil leaves, torn

Instructions:
1. Preheat the oven to 500°F.
2. Use a foil when lining a rimmed baking sheet, then set aside.
3. Put a tablespoon of canola oil in a large heavy-bottomed pan placed over high heat.
4. Sprinkle evenly half of the pepper and salt over the fish filets.
5. Cook the filets in the pan for 4 minutes until the sides are golden brown.
6. Transfer the filets, with seared sides up, onto the prepared baking sheet.
7. Put it in the oven and cook the filet for about 4 minutes or until you get the degree of doneness that you prefer.
8. Return the skillet to the stove, and add the remaining canola oil.
9. Add the shallots and sauté for a couple of minutes. Season with the remaining salt and pepper.

10. Add the cherry tomatoes and 1/3 cup basil. Cook until the tomatoes are soft, for about 2 minutes.

11. Add the balsamic vinegar. Stir and cook for about a minute.

12. Transfer the filets to a serving dish and top with the balsamic vinegar-tomato mixture. Garnish with the remaining basil.

13. Serve and enjoy while hot.

Chia Seed and Strawberry Pudding

Ingredients:
- 1 cup strawberries, thinly sliced
- 3 tbsp. chia seeds
- 1 cup soy beverage, unsweetened and fortified

Instructions:
1. To create pudding, combine the soy beverage and chia seeds.
2. Refrigerate the mixture for half an hour. Stir the mixture every 5 minutes to prevent the chia seeds from sticking together.
3. As an alternative, blend the soy beverage and chia seeds in a food processor and let it chill in the refrigerator.
4. Slice strawberries lengthwise.
5. Pour chilled pudding into 2 glasses. Place the strawberry slices on top.
6. Serve and enjoy your pudding.

Spinach Omelet

Ingredients:
- 2 egg whites
- 1 egg
- 1/2 cup fresh spinach

Instructions:
1. Put together beaten egg and egg whites, whilst forming a "pocket-like" shape.
2. Load the pocket with spinach. Cook until the spinach is wilted. Season with salt and pepper.
3. Serve immediately.

Barley and Chicken Soup

Ingredients:
- 4 cups vegetable broth
- 4 cups chicken broth
- 2-1/2 lb. chicken breast, cubed, bone and skin removed
- 2 cups butternut squash, peeled and cubed
- 2 cups yellow summer squash
- 2 cups cubed zucchini squash
- 1 cup white onion, diced
- 1 cup broccoli florets
- 8 oz. fresh mushrooms, chopped
- 1 cup barley
- 2 cups water
- 1 tbsp. garlic, minced
- 1 whole bay leaf
- 1/4 tsp. sea salt
- 1/4 tsp. ground black pepper

Instructions:
1. Pour the water, vegetable broth, and chicken broth in a large pot.
2. Add the chicken cubes, onion, garlic, bay leaf, salt, and black pepper.
3. Using medium-high heat, bring the contents of the pot to a boil.
4. Reduce the heat to low. Simmer for an hour.
5. Add the barley, broccoli, butternut squash, yellow summer squash, zucchini, and mushrooms into the pot.
6. Bring back to a boil.

7. Lower it to a simmer for about 60 to 120 minutes, or until vegetables have achieved your desired texture.

8. Transfer into a serving bowl immediately.

Bean Soup and Greens

Ingredients:
- 3 garlic cloves, minced
- 1 onion, diced
- 1 tbsp. coconut oil
- 2 tsp. freshly grated ginger
- 1 tsp. allspice
- 1 tsp. dried thyme
- 1-2 pcs. habanero or Scotch bonnet peppers, minced
- 1/2 tsp. black pepper
- 1/2 tsp. ground cinnamon
- 2 cups vegetable broth
- 14 oz.-can fire roasted tomatoes
- 14 oz.-can light coconut milk
- 14 oz.-can black beans, drained and rinsed
- 2 cans 14 oz. red kidney beans, drained and rinsed
- 1-1/2 tbsp. organic brown sugar
- 2 tbsp. lime juice
- 1 lb. collard greens, destemmed and torn into 1-2-inch pieces
- salt

Instructions:
1. In a pot over medium heat, heat the coconut for about a minute or two.
2. Add onion and cook for about 5 minutes. Stir until soft and translucent.
3. Stir in the ginger, garlic, and pepper. Cook for another minute until fragrant.
4. Add in the thyme, black pepper, allspice, and cinnamon. Stir.

5. Pour in the broth and coconut milk, followed by the beans and tomatoes.

6. Adjust the heat to high and leave the soup to boil.

7. Reduce the heat for simmering without the cover, until the beans soften, about 10 minutes.

8. To make a thicker soup, blend a small amount of the soup using a conventional or an immersion blender.

9. Throw in the collard greens upon serving.

<u>Cherry-Coconut Porridge</u>

Ingredients:
- fresh or frozen cherries
- 1-1/2 cups oats
- 4 tbsp. of chia seeds
- 3 tbsp. of raw cacao
- 3-4 cups coconut milk
- a pinch of stevia
- coconut shavings
- dark chocolate shavings
- maple syrup

Instructions:
1. Combine oats, cacao, Stevia, and coconut milk in a small saucepan.
2. Boil over medium heat. Simmer until the oats are well-cooked.
3. Pour into a bowl. Top with cherries, coconut shavings, maple syrup, and dark chocolate shavings.

Squash and Spinach Medley

Ingredients:
- 1 butternut squash, deseeded and sliced lengthwise
- 1 handful fresh baby spinach
- 2 tbsp. oil
- 1/4 tsp. sea salt
- 1-1/2 cups bone broth
- 1/2 tsp. Braggs Liquid Aminos
- 1 beet, sliced
- 2 tbsp. cashew yogurt

Instructions:
1. Preheat the oven to 425°F. Line a baking sheet with foil.
2. Brush 2 teaspoons of oil onto each half of the butternut squash. Season with salt.
3. Place each half on the baking sheet, flesh side down.
4. Place inside the oven and bake for 30 minutes until the flesh is soft.
5. Scoop the flesh out and place on a high speed blender. Add in baby spinach and bone broth. Puree until a smooth consistency is achieved.
6. Season with Braggs liquid Aminos.
7. Garnish with beets and yogurt.
8. Serve and enjoy.

Grilled Eggplant Salad

Ingredients:
- 4 small eggplants, sliced into circles and pressed dry with paper towels
- salt
- olive oil
- 1 cup beluga lentils, soaked overnight then rinsed and drained
- 1 tbsp. za'atar
- 1/4 cup golden raisins or currants
- 1/4 cup pine nuts, toasted
- 1 cup packed fresh herbs of mint, parsley, and dill
- 1 lemon, juice and zest
- black pepper
- salt

For the home blend za'atar:
- 1/4 cup sesame seeds, toasted
- 1/4 cup sumac
- 1/2 tsp. sea salt
- 1 tbsp. dried marjoram
- 2 tbsp. dried thyme

Instructions:
1. In a bowl, combine all the home blend ingredients. Mix well.
2. Transfer it to an airtight jar.
3. Place the eggplant in a colander and sprinkle generously with sea salt.
4. Set aside for half an hour to one, flipping over now and then.

5. Put the lentils in a large pot with 4 cups of water.

6. Bring to a boil, then reduce to a simmer for 20 minutes, until the lentils are cooked.

7. Preheat the barbecue or grill pan to medium-high heat.

8. Brush the sides of the eggplant generously with olive oil and sprinkle with za'atar.

9. Place on a grill and flip after 5 minutes, then cook for another 5 to 7 minutes.

10. Brush with extra olive oil if it looks dry.

11. Eggplant is done when the meaty center is soft and tender.

12. Toss the cooked lentils with all the herbs, raisins, and toasted pine nuts.

13. Season with salt and pepper.

14. Dress with a little olive oil and fresh lemon juice.

15. Add the grilled eggplant on top. Add a dash of extra za'atar and lemon zest.

Black Beans and Rice

Ingredients:
- 1 tsp. olive oil
- 1-1/2 cups vegetable broth, low-sodium
- 1 onion, chopped
- 1 tsp. ground cumin
- 1 garlic clove, minced
- 1/4 tsp. cayenne pepper
- 3/4 cup uncooked white rice
- 3-1/2 cups black beans in a can, drained

Instructions:
1. Pour olive oil into a stockpot over medium heat.
2. Sauté the onion and garlic in the heated stockpot for about 4 minutes.
3. Add the rice and cook for a couple more minutes.
4. Add the vegetable broth. Boil.
5. Lower the heat and cook for 20 minutes.
6. Add the black beans and the rest of the spices.
7. Serve while hot.

Mediterranean Tuna Salad

Ingredients:
- 1 5-oz. can Genova Yellowfin Tuna packed in olive oil
- a handful of watercress, rinsed and dried
- a handful of fresh green beans
- 1/2 cup canned black beans
- about 10 cherry tomatoes
- 1/2 cup canned garbanzo beans
- • 3 or 4 radishes, sliced paper-thin
- 1/2 cup canned cannellini beans
- basil leaves
- 1/2 cup canned red kidney beans
- lemon wedges
- fresh tarragon sprigs
- fresh thyme sprigs

For the tarragon vinaigrette:
- 2 tbsp. fresh tarragon, destemmed
- 2 tbsp. champagne vinegar or mild white vinegar
- 1 tsp. grainy Dijon mustard
- 1/4 tsp. salt
- 4 tbsp. olive oil
- 1/4 tsp. black pepper, freshly cracked

Instructions:
1. Blanch the green beans by dropping them in boiling water for 1-2 minutes.
2. Drain and quickly immerse in a bowl of ice water. Leave until the beans are cold. Drain and pat dry after.

3. Finely pulse the tarragon using a food processor or blender.

4. Add the rest of the vinaigrette ingredients and proceed to pulse until pureed.

5. On a plate, place some watercress in the center. Put tuna on top of it.

6. Rinse the beans and arrange them around the plate.

7. Add the green beans and tomato, followed by the radishes, fresh herbs, and lemon wedges.

8. Drizzle the vinaigrette on the salad upon serving.

Chicken Seafood Paella

Ingredients:
- 6 chicken thighs, skinless
- 3 cups Arborio rice
- 6 pcs. each of seafood ingredients: mussels, scallops, and clams of choice
- 2 ham hocks
- 2 cups seafood stock
- 4 tbsp. cooking oil, divided
- 1 cup carrots, chopped roughly
- 1 cup red bell pepper, diced
- 1 cup celery, roughly chopped
- 1 lb. Mexican style chorizo
- 1 cup apple cider vinegar
- 1 tbsp. saffron mixed with 1 cup water, steeped for 3 minutes
- salt
- black pepper
- 1/2 cup scallions, diced, for garnish

Instructions:
1. Pour 2 tablespoons of oil into a large stockpot placed over high heat.
2. Add ham hocks and chicken and cook until both thighs are evenly brown on each side.
3. Transfer chicken to a plate and set aside.
4. Continue cooking ham hocks. Add carrots and celery. Sauté for 7 minutes.
5. Deglaze by pouring white wine then decrease by half.

6. Pour seafood stock, around 2 quarts of water, and saffron mixture. Simmer to reduce liquid by half for 2 hours.

7. Once done, strain broth and simmer over low heat.

8. Heat the remaining oil in a paella pan.

9. Sauté chorizo, remaining onion slices, and red bell pepper. Cook until translucent without browning onions.

10. Add rice and season with salt and freshly ground black pepper according to preference.

11. Stir until rice grains are coated with oil.

12. Set rice around the pan to level then pour a cup of stock at a time without stirring.

13. Check if the rice is al dente or almost fully cooked then add the seafood ingredients and chicken thigh.

14. Cover seafood with rice to cook. Add the last cup of broth then cover the pan tightly.

15. Remove from heat and let paella sit for 15 minutes or until newly added ingredients are cooked.

16. Serve and enjoy while hot.

Cod Burger

Instructions:
- 1/3 cup cracked wheat
- 1-1/2 lb. cod
- 1 tsp. lemon juice
- canola oil cooking spray
- 1-1/2 cups cooked white beans, dry or canned, no salt added, rinsed and drained
- 1/2 cup chopped parsley
- 1/2 tsp. salt
- freshly ground black pepper, to taste
- 2 tsp. olive oil

Instructions:
1. Place cracked wheat in a bowl. Cover with 1/3 cup of boiling water. Let sit until water is absorbed, about 10 minutes.
2. Preheat the oven to 375°F.
3. Place cod on a baking dish, coat with lemon juice and vegetable oil cooking spray.
4. Cook until the fish starts to flake with the center still translucent, approximately 7 minutes.
5. Purée white beans in a blender or food processor.
6. Remove fish from the oven, let cool, and flake into a large bowl.
7. Add cracked wheat, beans, parsley, pepper, and salt. Hand mix everything.
8. Form into burger patties. This can make about four.
9. Over medium heat, coat a heavy-bottomed skillet with olive oil.

10. Fry burgers until each side is brown, about 4 minutes on one side.

Conclusion

Ehlers-Danlos Syndrome is a condition that affects people differently, not only physically but also emotionally and psychologically. People who have them have to learn how to live with chronic pain, changing their routines to adapt to their new lives. For some, their lives drastically change when their symptoms start to show and especially when they get diagnosed. Usually, even the most mundane things are affected by this condition.

They usually get fatigued easily, their actions and movements are limited by their condition, and even their surroundings could greatly affect their disposition simply because of how limiting the condition and its symptoms can be. It's always hard to explain this type of situation to other people who don't know them personally or those who don't understand the condition.

However, all these don't necessarily mean that people with EDS can't enjoy life anymore when they're diagnosed with this condition. There are ways to manage it and its symptoms to, at the very least, help the patient somehow live their life in the best way possible, even if there are limitations.

Managing Ehler-Danlos syndrome can be very challenging, not only for the diagnosed person but also for their family and friends. That's why proper support from the family, friends, and doctors of the person who has EDS is very important. While these simple suggestions to manage Ehlers-Danlos syndrome aren't exactly the cure for the condition, these may be beneficial in helping the patient improve their well-being.

References

Eccles, J. A., Beacher, F. D. C., Gray, M. A., Jones, C. L., Minati, L., Harrison, N. A., & Critchley, H. D. (2012). Brain structure and joint hypermobility: Relevance to the expression of psychiatric symptoms. British Journal of Psychiatry, 200(6), 508–509. https://doi.org/10.1192/bjp.bp.111.092460.

Ehlers-danlos syndrome: Symptoms, causes, treatments. (n.d.). Cleveland Clinic. Retrieved August 25, 2022, from https://my.clevelandclinic.org/health/diseases/17813-ehlers-danlos-syndrome.

Palomo-Toucedo, I., Leon-Larios, F., Reina-Bueno, M., Vázquez-Bautista, M., Munuera-Martínez, P., & Domínguez-Maldonado, G. (2020). Psychosocial influence of ehlers–danlos syndrome in daily life of patients: A qualitative study. International Journal of Environmental Research and Public Health, 17(17), 6425. https://doi.org/10.3390/ijerph17176425.

PhD, E. M. (n.d.). Ehlers-danlos syndrome and diet—What you need to know. Retrieved August 25, 2022, from https://ehlersdanlosnews.com/health-insights/low-sodium-diet-for-eds/.

Self management – the ehlers-danlos support uk. (n.d.). Retrieved August 25, 2022, from https://www.ehlers-danlos.org/what-is-eds/information-on-eds/self-management/.

The types of eds. (n.d.). The Ehlers Danlos Society. Retrieved August 25, 2022, from https://www.ehlers-danlos.com/eds-types/.

UC Davis Health, D. of A. and P. M. (n.d.). Division of Pain Medicine: UC Davis Medical Center. Division of Pain Medicine

| UC Davis Medical Center. Retrieved August 25, 2022, from https://health.ucdavis.edu/pain/.

What are the ehlers-danlos syndromes? (n.d.). The Ehlers Danlos Society. Retrieved August 25, 2022, from https://www.ehlers-danlos.com/what-is-eds/.

www.ingramcontent.com/pod-product-compliance
Ingram Content Group UK Ltd.
Pitfield, Milton Keynes, MK11 3LW, UK
UKHW021515290925

8129UKWH00036B/478

9 781087 934525